ACID REFLUX

COOKBOOK

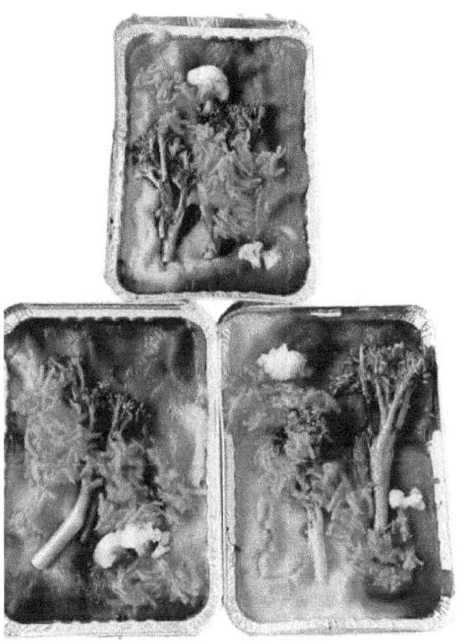

A Culinary Approach to Digestive Health

Ava Harding

All rights reserved. No part of this publication may be reproduced, distributed, or transmitted in any form or by any means, including photocopying, recording, or other electronic or mechanic methods, without the prior written permission of the publisher, except in the case of brief quotations embodied in critical reviews and certain other noncommercial uses permitted by copyright law.

Copyright © by Ava Harding 2023

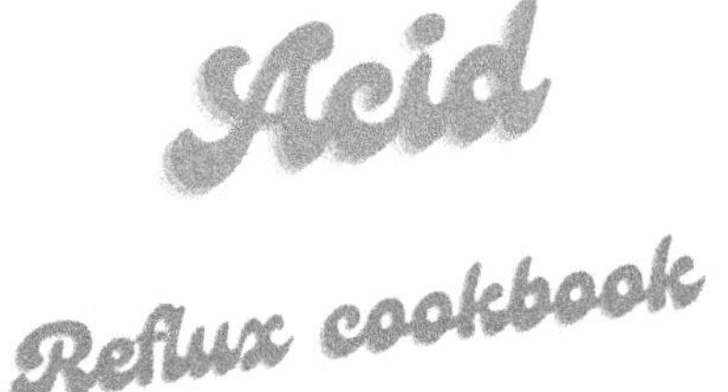

TABLE OF CONTENTS

INTRODUCTION

Comfort had suffered from acid reflux for years, and mealtimes had become a source of pain and irritation. Her chronic heartburn and indigestion had made it difficult for her to enjoy her favorite foods. That's when a friend recommended an acid reflux cookbook to her.

Comfort decided to give it a shot despite her reservations. The influence it had on her life shocked her. The cookbook included a variety of delicious, quick, and simple meals that were specifically designed to be pleasant on her stomach.

These meals not only delighted her taste senses, but they also alleviated her acid reflux symptoms. She could finally eat without worry or discomfort.

Comfort found that following the acid reflux cookbook had improved not just her health but also her general enjoyment of life. She could finally eat meals with family and friends, brightening and enhancing her days.

Acid reflux is a common disorder in which stomach acid runs back into the esophagus. Gastroesophageal reflux disease (GERD) is another name for it. This backflow of stomach acid can induce esophageal irritation and inflammation, resulting in a variety of symptoms. Understanding acid reflux forms, causes, symptoms, and preventive strategies is critical for optimal management of this problem.

Types of Acid Reflux

1. **Non-Erosive Reflux Disease (NERD):** This type of acid reflux is distinguished by usual symptoms and the absence of apparent esophageal damage during endoscopy.

2. **Reflux Esophagitis:** This type is distinguished by esophageal lining irritation and destruction as a result of prolonged exposure to stomach acid.

3. **Barrett's Esophagus:** In some situations, chronic acid reflux can cause alterations in the esophageal lining, raising the risk of esophageal cancer.

Causes of Acid Reflux

1. **Hiatal Hernia:** A disorder in which a portion of the stomach protrudes into the chest cavity, increasing the risk of acid reflux.

2. **Weakened Lower Esophageal Sphincter (LES):** The LES is a muscular band that connects the esophagus to the stomach. As it deteriorates, stomach acid might leak back into the esophagus.

3. **Dietary Factors:** Acid reflux can be triggered by acidic, fatty, or spicy foods, as well as excessive coffee and alcohol consumption.

4. **Obesity:** Excess weight exerts strain on the abdomen, causing stomach acid to back up.

5. **Pregnancy:** Acid reflux can be exacerbated by hormonal changes during pregnancy as well as the pressure exerted by the enlarging uterus.

Symptoms of Acid Reflux

1. **Heartburn:** A burning sensation in the chest, usually after eating or lying down.

2. **Regurgitation:** The passage of stomach contents into the mouth.

3. **Chest Pain:** Discomfort or pain in the chest, which is commonly misinterpreted as a heart attack.

4. **Difficulty Swallowing:** This is known as dysphagia, and it can arise as a result of esophageal injury.

5. **Chronic Cough:** A persistent cough, particularly at night, maybe a sign.

Complications of Acid Reflux

Untreated acid reflux, which is additionally known as gastroesophageal reflux disease (GERD), can cause a variety of issues that affect both the esophagus and overall health. Chronic esophageal exposure to stomach acid can result in:

1. **Esophagitis:** Inflammation of the esophagus can cause discomfort, problems with swallowing, and scarring.

2. **Barrett's Esophagus:** Long-term acid exposure can cause alterations in the cells that line the esophagus, raising the risk of esophageal cancer.

3. **Stricture:** Repeated inflammation can cause the esophagus to constrict, making swallowing difficult.

4. **Respiratory Issues:** Stomach acid can enter the throat and airways, causing or aggravating asthma, persistent cough, and pneumonia.

5. **Dental Problems:** Acid erosion can damage tooth enamel, resulting in cavities and tooth discomfort.

6. **Esophageal Ulcers:** Due to extended exposure to stomach acid, open sores in the esophagus may form, causing pain and possibly bleeding.

7. **Aspiration Pneumonia:** In severe situations, the contents of the stomach may be aspirated into the lungs, increasing the risk of pneumonia.

Preventive Measures For Acid Reflux

1. Lifestyle Modifications:

- Dietary Changes: Avoiding foods like citrus, chocolate, and caffeine.

- Weight Management: Maintaining a healthy weight to relieve abdominal pressure.

- Elevating the Head of the Bed: Sleeping with your upper body elevated to keep stomach acid from flowing up into your esophagus.

2. Medications:

- Antacids: By neutralizing stomach acid, it provides immediate comfort.

- H2 Blockers: Reducing stomach acid production.

- Proton Pump Inhibitors (PPIs): Blocking acid production over a longer amount of time.

3. Behavioral Changes:

- Eating Habits: Taking smaller meals and avoiding lying down just after eating.

- Quitting Smoking: Cigarette smoking weakens the LES, which contributes to acid reflux.

- Stress Management: Stress can aggravate symptoms, so adopting stress-relieving hobbies is good.

4. Surgery:

In severe cases, when lifestyle changes and drugs are inadequate, surgical intervention to strengthen the LES or repair hiatal hernias may be considered.

30 ACID REFLUX RECIPES

Baked Chicken Meatballs

Ingredients:

- One-pound ground chicken

- 1/4 cup of breadcrumbs

- 1/4 cup of grated Parmesan cheese

- 1/4 cup of finely chopped onion

- Two cloves garlic, minced

- One egg

- One teaspoon of Italian seasoning

- Salt and pepper to taste well

- The Marinara sauce for dipping (optional)

Preparation Method:

1. Preheat your oven to 375°F (190°C).

2. In a mixing bowl, combine the ground chicken, breadcrumbs, Parmesan cheese, chopped onion, minced garlic, egg, Italian seasoning, salt, and pepper.

3. Form the mixture into meatballs and place them on a baking sheet lined with parchment paper.

4. Bake in a preheated oven for 20-25 minutes, or until the meatballs are cooked through and golden brown.

5. Serve with marinara sauce for dipping, if preferred.

Summer Squash Pasta Skillet

Ingredients:

- Eight ounces pasta (your choice)

- Two tablespoons of olive oil

- One onion, chopped

- Two cloves garlic, minced

- Two summer squash, sliced

- One cup of cherry tomatoes, halved

- Salt and pepper to taste well

- Fresh basil leaves for garnish

- Grated Parmesan cheese (optional)

Preparation Method:

1. Prepare the pasta according to the package directions, drain it, and set it aside.

2. Heat the olive oil in a large skillet over medium heat flame. Sauté the chopped onion and minced garlic until it is softened.

3. Toss in the cut summer squash and halved cherry tomatoes. Cook for 5-7 minutes, or until the vegetables are tender.

4. Season to taste it with salt and pepper to taste well.

5. Stir in the cooked spaghetti to mix.

6. If wanted, garnish with fresh basil leaves and grated Parmesan cheese.

Chicken Tenders with Sesame-crusted

Ingredients:

- One-pound chicken tenders

- 1/2 cup of sesame seeds

- 1/4 cup of breadcrumbs

- 1/4 cup of flour

- One egg, beaten

- Salt and pepper to taste well

- Cooking spray

Preparation Method:

1. Line a baking sheet with parchment paper for optimum results and preheat the oven to a temperature of 375°F (190°C).

2. Combine sesame seeds, breadcrumbs, flour, salt, and pepper in a shallow plate.

3. Coat each chicken tender with the sesame seed mixture after dipping it in the beaten egg.

4. Arrange the coated chicken tenders on the prepared baking sheet.

5. Spray the tenders lightly with cooking spray to help them crisp up.

6. Bake for 20 to 25 minutes, or until the chicken is thoroughly cooked and the coating is golden brown.

Easy Veggie Quesadillas

Ingredients:

- Four large flour tortillas

- One cup of shredded cheese (your preferred choice)

- One cup of mixed vegetables (bell peppers, onions, mushrooms, etc.), sliced

- One tablespoon of olive oil

- Salt and pepper to taste well

- The salsa and sour cream for dipping (optional)

Preparation Method:

1. Heat the olive oil in a large skillet over medium heat flame. Sauté the cut vegetables until they are soft. Season with salt and pepper to allow it to taste well.

2. In the griddle, place a tortilla and top with shredded cheese.

3. Pile some sautéed vegetables on top of the cheese.

4. Place another tortilla on top and gently press down.

5. Cook the tortillas for a few minutes on each side, or until brown and the cheese is melted.

6. Continue with the rest of the tortillas and filling.

7. Serve in wedges with salsa and sour cream, if desired.

Sheet Pan Cashew Chicken

Ingredients:

- One and a half pounds of boneless, skinless chicken breasts, diced

- One cup of broccoli florets

- One cup of bell peppers, sliced

- 1/2 cup cashews

- Two tablespoons of olive oil

- Three tablespoons of soy sauce

- Two tablespoons of honey

- Two cloves garlic, minced

- Salt and pepper to taste well

- Cooked rice for serving

Preparation Method:

1. Line a baking sheet with parchment paper for optimum results and preheat the oven to a temperature of 425°F (220°C).

2. Combine the olive oil, soy sauce, honey, minced garlic, salt, and pepper in a mixing bowl.

3. Arrange the chicken pieces, broccoli florets, and bell pepper slices on the baking sheet that has been prepared.

4. Drizzle the chicken and vegetables with the soy sauce mixture.

5. Toss everything together until evenly coated, then spread out in a single layer.

6. Sprinkle with cashews on top.

7. Bake for 15-20 minutes, or until the chicken is thoroughly cooked and the vegetables are soft.

8. Serve with cooked rice.

Roasted Vegetable Lasagna

Ingredients:

- Nine lasagna noodles, cooked and drained

- Two cups of ricotta cheese

- One egg

- One cup of grated mozzarella cheese

- 1/2 cup of grated Parmesan cheese

- One zucchini, sliced

- One red bell pepper, sliced

- One yellow bell pepper, sliced

- One onion, sliced

- Two cups of marinara sauce

- Salt and pepper to taste well

- Fresh basil leaves for garnish (optional)

Preparation Method:

1. Preheat your oven to 375°F (190°C).

2. Combine ricotta cheese, egg, grated mozzarella, and grated Parmesan in a mixing basin. Season with salt and pepper to allow it to taste well.

3. Spread a thin layer of marinara sauce in a large baking dish.

4. Top the sauce with 3 cooked lasagna noodles.

5. Spread half of the ricotta mixture over the noodles.

6. Layer half of the sliced veggies on top of the ricotta mixture.

7. Repeat with another layer of noodles, the remaining ricotta mixture, and the remaining vegetables.

8. Add a final layer of noodles and top with marinara sauce.

9. If preferred, top with more mozzarella and Parmesan cheese.

10. Bake for 30-35 minutes, or until the lasagna is bubbling and the cheese is brown, in a preheated oven.

11. Before serving it, garnish it with fresh basil leaves.

Maple BBQ Salmon

Ingredients:

- Four salmon fillets

- 1/4 cup of maple syrup

- Two tablespoons of barbecue sauce

- One tablespoon of soy sauce

- One teaspoon of Dijon mustard

- Salt and pepper to taste well

Preparation Method:

1. Preheat your grill to medium-high heat flame.

2. Whisk together maple syrup, barbecue sauce, soy sauce, Dijon mustard, salt, and pepper in a mixing bowl.

3. Drizzle the maple BBQ sauce over the salmon fillets.

4. Grill the salmon for 4-5 minutes per side, or until it flakes easily with a fork and develops grill marks.

Grilled Tahini-Glazed Salmon with Cucumber Noodles

Ingredients:

- Four salmon fillets

- 1/4 cup of tahini

- Two tablespoons of soy sauce

- Two tablespoons of honey

- One tablespoon of rice vinegar

- Two cloves garlic, minced

- Two cucumbers, spiralized into noodles

- Green chopped onions and sesame seeds as a garnish.

Preparation Method:

1. Preheat your grill to medium-high heat flame.

2. Combine tahini, soy sauce, honey, rice vinegar, and minced garlic in a mixing bowl.

3. Drizzle the tahini glaze over the salmon fillets.

4. Grill the salmon for 4-5 minutes per side, or until it reaches the desired amount of doneness.

5. While the salmon is frying, cook the cucumber noodles in a skillet until they are barely soft.

6. Arrange the grilled salmon over cucumber noodles and top with sesame seeds and green onions.

30-Minute Chicken Stir Fry

Ingredients:

- Cut into bite-sized pieces, one pound of boneless, skinless chicken breasts

- Two cups of mixed vegetables (bell peppers, broccoli, carrots, etc.), sliced

- Two tablespoons of vegetable oil

- 1/4 cup of soy sauce

- Two tablespoons of honey

- One tablespoon of cornstarch

- One teaspoon of minced garlic

- Cooked rice for serving

Preparation Method:

1. In a large skillet, heat the vegetable oil over medium-high heat flame.

2. Stir-fry the chicken pieces until they are cooked through and no longer pink.

3. Remove the chicken from the skillet and set it aside.

4. Add the mixed vegetables to the same skillet and stir-fry for a few minutes, or until tender-crisp.

5. Combine soy sauce, honey, cornstarch, and minced garlic in a mixing dish.

6. Return the cooked chicken to the skillet, pour the sauce over it, and mix to coat.

7. Cook for another 2-3 minutes, or until it is thickened.

8. Toss the chicken stir fry with the cooked rice.

Coconut Curry Chicken with Peanut Dipping Sauce

Ingredients:

- Four boneless, skinless chicken breasts

- One can (Fourteen ounces) coconut milk

- Two tablespoons of red curry paste

- Two tablespoons of peanut butter

- One tablespoon of soy sauce

- One tablespoon of honey

- One tablespoon of lime juice

- Chopped cilantro and chopped peanuts for garnish

Preparation Method:

1. Heat the coconut milk in a large skillet over medium-high heat flame until it begins to simmer.

2. Combine the red curry paste, peanut butter, soy sauce, honey, and lime juice in a mixing bowl. Continue to cook it and whisk the sauce until it thickens.

3. Place the chicken breasts in the skillet and cook for 15-20 minutes, or until it is cooked through.

4. Before serving it, garnish with chopped cilantro and chopped peanuts.

Creamy White Sauce Chicken Enchiladas

Ingredients:

- Two cups of cooked chicken, shredded

- Eight small flour tortillas

- Two cups of shredded Monterey Jack cheese

- Two tablespoons of butter

- Two tablespoons of all-purpose flour

- 1 1/2 cups of chicken broth

- One cup of sour cream

- One can of diced green chilies (Four ounces)

- Salt and pepper to taste well

Preparation Method:

1. Preheat your oven to 350°F (175°C).

2. Combine shredded chicken and one cup shredded cheese in a large mixing basin. Roll the mixture into tortillas and set them on a baking tray that has been buttered.

3. Melt butter in a saucepan over medium heat. Cook for a minute, stirring constantly, until the flour is lightly browned.

4. Whisk in the chicken broth gradually and boil until the mixture thickens.

5. Remove from the fire and toss in the sour cream, diced green chilies, salt, and pepper.

6. Spoon the sauce over the enchiladas and top with the remaining 1 cup shredded cheese.

7. Bake it for 20-25 minutes, or until the enchiladas are heated through and the cheese is melted and bubbling, in a preheated oven.

10-Minute Blackened Tilapia

Ingredients:

- Four tilapia fillets

- Two tablespoons of blackening seasoning

- Two tablespoons of olive oil

- Lemon wedges for serving

Preparation Method:

1. In a large skillet over medium-high heat flame, heat the olive oil.

2. Evenly rub the blackening seasoning over both sides of the tilapia fillets.

3. Cook the fillets for 3-4 minutes per side, or until the salmon flakes easily with a fork and has a browned crust.

4. Garnish it with lemon wedges for squeezing on top.

Teriyaki Shrimp Sushi Bowl

Ingredients:

- One cup of sushi rice

- One cup of cooked, peeled, and deveined shrimp

- 1/4 cup of teriyaki sauce

- 1/2 avocado, sliced

- 1/2 cucumber, thinly sliced

- 1/2 carrot, julienned

- One nori seaweed sheet, crumbled

- Sesame seeds for garnish (optional)

Preparation Method:

1. Prepare sushi rice according to package directions and set it aside to cool.

2. Combine cooked shrimp and teriyaki sauce in a mixing bowl.

3. Layer sushi rice, teriyaki shrimp, avocado, cucumber, carrot, and crumbled nori sheet in a bowl.

4. If preferred, top it with sesame seeds for extra taste.

Parmesan Orzo with Mushrooms and Spinach

Ingredients:

- One cup of orzo pasta

- Two cups of fresh spinach

- One cup of mushrooms, sliced

- 1/2 cup of grated Parmesan cheese

- Two cloves garlic, minced

- Two tablespoons of olive oil

- Salt and pepper to taste well

Preparation Method:

1. Prepare orzo pasta according to its package directions. Set it aside after draining.

2. Heat the olive oil in a large skillet over medium heat flame. Incorporate the minced garlic and cut mushrooms. Cook until the mushrooms are soft.

3. Cook it until the spinach has wilted in the skillet used.

4. Fold in the cooked orzo and Parmesan cheese. Toss until the cheese is melted and everything is properly incorporated.

5. Season it to taste well with salt and pepper and serve it.

Cheesy Broccoli Loaded Baked Potatoes

Ingredients:

- Four russet potatoes

- Two cups of broccoli florets, steamed

- One cup of shredded cheddar cheese

- 1/2 cup of sour cream

- Two tablespoons of butter

- Salt and pepper to taste well

Preparation Method:

1. Preheat the oven to 400°F (200°C).

2. Scrub the potatoes and pierce them with a fork. Bake it for 45-60 minutes, or until it is tender, in a preheated oven.

3. Slit the tops of the potatoes and fluff the insides with a fork.

4. Arrange the steamed broccoli florets, cheddar cheese, a dollop of sour cream, and a dab of butter on top of each potato.

5. Season it to taste well with salt and pepper and serve it while still hot.

Butternut Squash Mac and Cheese

Ingredients:

- Eight ounces of elbow macaroni

- Two cups of butternut squash puree

- One cup of shredded sharp cheddar cheese

- 1/2 cup of milk (either dairy or plant-based)

- Two tablespoons of butter

- 1/4 teaspoon of nutmeg

- Salt and pepper to taste well

Preparation Method:

1. Prepare the elbow macaroni according to its package directions. Set it aside after draining.

2. Heat the butternut squash puree, milk, butter, and nutmeg in a skillet over medium heat flame, stirring it constantly.

3. Stir in the shredded cheddar cheese and simmer until the cheese melts and the sauce thickens.

4. Combine the cooked macaroni and the butternut squash cheese sauce in a mixing bowl.

5. Season it to taste well with salt and pepper and serve it.

Quinoa Crusted Salmon

Ingredients:

- Four salmon fillets

- One cup of cooked quinoa

- 1/4 cup of grated Parmesan cheese

- One teaspoon of dried thyme

- One teaspoon of paprika

- Salt and pepper to taste well

- Olive oil for brushing

Preparation Method:

1. Preheat the oven to 375°F (190°C) and line the baking sheet with the parchment paper.

2. Combine cooked quinoa, grated Parmesan cheese, dried thyme, paprika, salt, and pepper in a mixing dish.

3. Brush the salmon fillets with olive oil, then press the quinoa mixture on top.

4. Bake the coated salmon fillets for 15-20 minutes, or until the salmon flakes easily with a fork, on the prepared baking sheet.

30-Minute Fall Veggie Pizza

Ingredients:

- One pizza dough (either store-bought or homemade)

- 1/2 cup of pizza sauce

- One cup of shredded mozzarella cheese

- 1/2 cup of roasted butternut squash cubes

- 1/2 cup of sautéed spinach

- 1/4 cup of caramelized onions

- 1/4 cup of crumbled goat cheese

- Fresh thyme leaves for garnish (optional)

Preparation Method:

1. Preheat your oven to the temperature recommended for your pizza dough (usually around 450°F or 230°C).

2. Place the pizza dough on a pizza stone or baking sheet and roll it out.

3. Evenly spread pizza sauce over the dough and top with shredded mozzarella cheese.

4. Add roasted butternut squash cubes, sautéed spinach, caramelized onions, and crumbled goat cheese on the pizza.

5. Bake for 12-15 minutes, or until the crust is brown and the cheese is bubbling, in a preheated oven.

6. If preferred, garnish it with fresh thyme leaves, slice, and serve your homemade fall vegetarian pizza.

Cheesy Chicken Pesto Spaghetti Squash

Ingredients:

- One medium spaghetti squash

- Two boneless, skinless chicken breasts

- 1/2 cup of pesto sauce

- One cup of shredded mozzarella cheese

- Salt and pepper to taste well

- Olive oil for cooking

Preparation Method:

1. Preheat your oven to 375°F (190°C).

2. Remove the seeds after slicing the spaghetti squash in half lengthwise.

3. Drizzle olive oil inside the squash halves and season it with salt and pepper.

4. Place the squash halves on a baking sheet cut-side down and bake for 30-40 minutes, or until the flesh is soft.

5. Season the chicken breasts with salt and pepper and sauté them in a skillet with olive oil until it is thoroughly done while the squash bakes.

6. Combine the cooked chicken with the pesto sauce.

7. When the squash is done, scrape the flesh into spaghetti-like strands with a fork.

8. Spoon the chicken and pesto mixture into each squash half, then top with shredded mozzarella cheese.

9. Return the squash halves to the oven and broil for a few minutes, or until the cheese is melted and bubbling.

10. Serve it immediately.

Mediterranean Farro Salad with Arugula and Chickpeas

Ingredients:

- One cup of Farro

- Two cups of water or vegetable broth

- One cup of canned, washed and drained chickpeas

- Two cups of arugula

- 1/2 cup of cherry tomatoes, halved

- Kalamata olives, cut and pitted, 1/4 cup

- 1/4 cup crumbled feta cheese

- Two tablespoons of extra-virgin olive oil

- Two tablespoons of lemon juice

- One clove garlic, minced

- Salt and pepper to taste well

Preparation Method:

1. Wash the farro in cool water. Combine the farro and water or vegetable broth in a saucepan. Bring it to a boil, then lower to a low heat, cover, and cook for 20-25 minutes, or until the farro is soft. Allow any surplus liquid to drain and cool.

2. Toss together the cooked farro, chickpeas, arugula, cherry tomatoes, Kalamata olives, and feta cheese in a large salad dish.

3. In a small bowl, combine the olive oil, lemon juice, garlic powder, salt, and pepper.

4. Toss the salad with the dressing to coat it.

5. Serve it chilled.

Green Goddess Chicken Salad Phyllo Cups

Ingredients:

- Two cups of cooked chicken, diced

- 1/2 cup of plain Greek yogurt

- 1/4 cup of mayonnaise

- Two tablespoons of fresh basil, chopped

- Two tablespoons of fresh parsley, chopped

- One tablespoon of fresh chives, chopped

- One tablespoon of fresh tarragon, chopped

- One clove garlic, minced

- Salt and pepper to taste well

- Phyllo cups (either store-bought or homemade)

Preparation Method:

1. In a mixing bowl, combine the diced chicken, Greek yogurt, mayonnaise, fresh herbs, minced garlic, salt, and pepper. Mix it until well combined.

2. Spoon the chicken salad mixture into the phyllo cups.

3. Serve it.

Seared Scallops with Acorn Squash Mash

Ingredients:

- Twelve large scallops

- Two halved acorn squashes, and seeds removed

- Two tablespoons of olive oil

- Salt and pepper to taste well

- Two tablespoons of butter

- Fresh thyme leaves for garnish (optional)

Preparation Method:

1. Preheat your oven to 400°F (200°C).

2. Drizzle olive oil over the acorn squash halves and season it with salt and pepper to taste well.

3. Place the squash halves on a baking sheet cut-side down and roast it for 40-50 minutes, or until the flesh is soft.

4. Season the scallops with salt and pepper while the squash roasts.

5. Melt butter in a pan over medium-high heat flame. Sear the scallops for 2-3 minutes per side, or until it is well browned and cooked through.

6. When the squash is finished cooking, scoop out the flesh and mash it with a fork or potato masher.

7. Arrange the cooked scallops on a bed of mashed acorn squash and sprinkle with fresh thyme leaves, if preferred.

One Pan Honey Mustard Chicken and Potatoes

Ingredients:

- Four boneless, skinless chicken breasts

- Four cups of baby potatoes, halved

- 1/4 cup of Dijon mustard

- Two tablespoons of honey

- Two tablespoons of olive oil

- One teaspoon of paprika

- One teaspoon of garlic powder

- Salt and pepper to taste well

- Fresh parsley for garnish (optional)

Preparation Method:

1. Preheat your oven to 400°F (200°C).

2. To make the honey mustard sauce, whisk together Dijon mustard, honey, olive oil, paprika, garlic powder, salt, and pepper in a mixing bowl.

3. Arrange the chicken breasts and baby potatoes, halved, on a large baking sheet or roasting pan.

4. Drizzle the honey mustard sauce over the chicken and potatoes, being careful to coat everything evenly.

5. Toss the potatoes to cover them evenly with the sauce.

6. Bake for 25-30 minutes, or until the chicken is cooked through and the potatoes are soft, in a preheated oven. Check that the chicken's internal temperature reaches 165°F (74°C).

7. Remove from the oven and, if wanted, sprinkle with fresh parsley.

8. Enjoy the delightful tastes of your one-pan honey mustard chicken and potatoes.

Mushroom Spinach White Pizza

Ingredients:

- One prepared pizza dough

- One cup ricotta cheese

- Two cups mozzarella cheese, shredded

- Two cups fresh spinach

- 1 1/2 cups mushrooms, thinly sliced

- Two cloves garlic, minced

- Olive oil for drizzling

- Salt and pepper to taste well

- Red pepper flakes for optional spice

Preparation Method:

1. Preheat your oven according to the directions on the pizza dough.

2. Roll out the pizza dough to the appropriate thickness and shape on a floured surface.

3. Combine the ricotta cheese, minced garlic, and a pinch of salt and pepper in a mixing bowl.

4. Evenly distribute the ricotta mixture over the pizza dough, leaving a border for the crust.

5. Top the ricotta mixture with shredded mozzarella cheese.

6. Evenly scatter fresh spinach leaves and sliced mushrooms over the cheese.

7. Drizzle a little olive oil over the pizza and season with salt and pepper to taste well.

8. If you want it hot, top it with red pepper flakes.

9. Bake for the time specified for your pizza dough, or until the crust is brown and the cheese is bubbling, in a preheated oven.

10. Take your homemade mushroom spinach white pizza out of the oven, slice it, and enjoy.

Apricot Chicken Thighs with Root Vegetables

Ingredients:

- Four bone-in, skin-on chicken thighs

- Two carrots, peeled and chopped

- Two parsnips, peeled and chopped

- Two sweet potatoes, peeled and chopped

- 1/2 cup of apricot preserves

- Two tablespoons of olive oil

- Two tablespoons of balsamic vinegar

- Two cloves garlic, minced

- Salt and pepper to taste well

- Fresh parsley for garnish (optional)

Preparation Method:

1. Preheat your oven to 375°F (190°C).

2. Combine apricot preserves, olive oil, balsamic vinegar, minced garlic, salt, and pepper in a mixing bowl.

3. In a large oven-proof dish or roasting pan, combine the chicken thighs, carrots, parsnips, and sweet potatoes.

4. Brush the apricot mixture over the chicken and vegetables to cover thoroughly.

5. Roast it for 45-50 minutes, or until the chicken is cooked through and the vegetables are soft, in a preheated oven.

6. Before serving, garnish it with fresh parsley if preferred.

Teriyaki Turkey Skillet with Vegetables

Ingredients:

- One-pound ground turkey

- Two cups of mixed vegetables; it can be bell peppers, broccoli, or carrots.

- 1/4 cup of teriyaki sauce

- Two tablespoons of soy sauce

- One tablespoon of sesame oil

- Two cloves garlic, minced

- One teaspoon of grated ginger

- Either Cooked rice or cauliflower rice for serving

Preparation Method:

1. Heat sesame oil in a large skillet over medium-high heat flame.

2. Cook until the ground turkey is browned, breaking it up with a spoon as it cooks.

3. Cook it for another minute, stirring in the minced garlic and grated ginger, until fragrant.

4. Stir in the mixed vegetables and simmer until they soften.

5. Stir in the teriyaki sauce and soy sauce to evenly coat the turkey and vegetables.

6. Cook for a few minutes more, or until the veggies are soft and the sauce has thickened.

7. Serve it with rice or cauliflower rice.

Banh Mi Bowls with Sticky Tofu

Ingredients:

- One block of extra-firm tofu, cubed

- 1/4 cup of soy sauce

- Two tablespoons of hoisin sauce

- One tablespoon of either honey or agave nectar

- Two cups of either cooked rice or rice noodles

- Sliced cucumbers, pickled carrots, and fresh cilantro for topping

- Sriracha sauce for added spice (optional)

Preparation Method:

1. Combine the soy sauce, hoisin sauce, and honey in a mixing dish. Combine it thoroughly.

2. Marinate the tofu cubes in the sauce for 15-20 minutes.

3. Melt the marinated tofu cubes in a nonstick skillet over medium-high heat flame. Cook until the outsides are sticky and somewhat crispy.

4. Put cooked rice or rice noodles in a bowl and assemble your banh mi bowls.

5. Garnish it with sticky tofu, sliced cucumbers, pickled carrots, fresh cilantro, and a drizzle of Sriracha sauce, if desired.

Green Pizza with Pesto, Feta, Artichokes, and Broccoli

Ingredients:

- One pizza dough (either store-bought or homemade)

- 1/2 cup of pesto sauce

- 1/2 cup of crumbled feta cheese

- Half a cup chopped marinated artichoke hearts

- 1 cup of either blanched or steamed broccoli florets

- Red pepper flakes for optional spice

Preparation Method:

1. Preheat your oven according to the directions on the pizza dough.

2. Roll out the pizza dough to the appropriate thickness and shape on a floured surface.

3. Evenly spread the pesto sauce over the pizza dough, leaving a boundary for the crust.

4. Top the pesto with crumbled feta cheese.

5. Evenly distribute chopped marinated artichoke hearts and blanched or steamed broccoli florets over the pie.

6. If you want it hot, top with red pepper flakes.

7. Bake for the time specified for your pizza dough, or until the crust is brown and the toppings are heated through.

8. Cut and serve your own green pizza!

Chicken Tortellini with Broccoli Bake

Ingredients:

- One-pound cheese tortellini

- Two cups of cooked chicken, diced

- Steamed or blanched, two cups of broccoli florets

- One and half cups of shredded mozzarella cheese

- 1/2 cup of grated Parmesan cheese

- One cup of Alfredo sauce

- 1/2 teaspoon of garlic powder

- Salt and pepper to taste well

- Fresh parsley for garnish (optional)

Preparation Method:

1. Preheat your oven to 375°F (190°C).

2. Prepare the cheese tortellini according to its package directions. Set it aside after draining.

3. Combine the cooked chicken, blanched broccoli florets, shredded mozzarella cheese, grated Parmesan cheese, Alfredo sauce, garlic powder, salt, and pepper in a large mixing dish.

4. Toss in the cooked tortellini and gently toss it to incorporate.

5. Pour the entire mixture into a greased baking dish.

6. Bake it for 20-25 minutes, or until the top is golden and bubbling, in a preheated oven.

7. Before serving it, garnish with fresh parsley if preferred.

Balsamic Chicken

Ingredients:

- Four boneless, skinless chicken breasts

- 1/4 cup of balsamic vinegar

- Two tablespoons of olive oil

- Two cloves garlic, minced

- One teaspoon of dried Italian seasoning

- Salt and pepper to taste well

- Fresh basil leaves for garnish (optional)

Preparation Method:

1. Whisk together the balsamic vinegar, olive oil, minced garlic, dried Italian seasoning, salt, and pepper in a mixing bowl.

2. Pour the balsamic marinade over the chicken breasts in a resealable plastic bag or shallow dish. Close the bag or cover the dish and leave it in the refrigerator for at least 30 minutes to marinate.

3. Heat a grill or grill pan over medium-high heat flame.

4. Remove the chicken from the marinade and grill for 6-8 minutes per side, or until cooked through and grill marks

appear. The internal temperature should be around 165°F (74°C).

5. Before serving it, garnish it with fresh basil leaves if desired.

MEAL PLAN

DAY 1:

- **Breakfast:** Coconut Curry Chicken with Peanut Dipping Sauce

- **Lunch:** Teriyaki Shrimp Sushi Bowl

- **Dinner:** Cheesy Broccoli Loaded Baked Potatoes

DAY 2

- **Breakfast:** Green Goddess Chicken Salad Phyllo Cups

- **Lunch:** Mushroom Spinach White Pizza

- **Dinner:** Teriyaki Turkey Skillet with Vegetables

DAY 3

- **Breakfast:** Baked Chicken Meatballs

- **Lunch:** Green Pizza with Pesto, Feta, Artichokes, and Broccoli

- **Dinner:** One Pan Honey Mustard Chicken and Potatoes

DAY 4

- **Breakfast:** Cheesy Chicken Pesto Spaghetti Squash

- **Lunch:** Apricot Chicken Thighs with Root Vegetables

- **Dinner:** Parmesan Orzo with Mushrooms and Spinach

DAY 5

- **Breakfast:** Quinoa Crusted Salmon

- **Lunch:** Chicken Tortellini with Broccoli Bake

- **Dinner:** Maple BBQ Salmon

DAY 6

- **Breakfast:** Mediterranean Farro Salad with Arugula and Chickpeas

- **Lunch:** Seared Scallops with Acorn Squash Mash

- **Dinner:** 30-Minute Chicken Stir Fry

DAY 7

- Breakfast: Grilled Tahini-Glazed Salmon with Cucumber Noodles

- **Lunch:** Banh Mi Bowls with Sticky Tofu

- **Dinner:** Creamy White Sauce Chicken Enchiladas

DAY 8

- **Breakfast:** 10-Minute Blackened Tilapia

- **Lunch:** Chicken Tenders with Sesame-crusted

- **Dinner:** Teriyaki Shrimp Sushi Bowl

DAY 9

- **Breakfast:** Easy Veggie Quesadillas

- **Lunch:** Roasted Vegetable Lasagna

- **Dinner:** Balsamic Chicken

DAY 10

- **Breakfast:** Butternut Squash Mac and Cheese

- **Lunch:** Sheet Pan Cashew Chicken

- **Dinner:** Chicken Tortellini with Broccoli Bake

Benefits of Following Acid Reflux Diet

Following an acid reflux diet can provide a number of key benefits, including symptom relief and improved general health. Here are some significant benefits:

1. **Reduced Heartburn:** Heartburn, the most prevalent symptom of acid reflux, can be reduced with a well-managed acid reflux diet. Avoiding trigger foods and making attentive decisions help to reduce this.

2. **Less Esophageal Irritation:** Acid reflux diet adjustments serve to reduce esophageal irritation and inflammation, lowering the risk of disorders such as esophagitis.

3. **Improved Sleep Quality:** Individuals can enhance their sleep quality by avoiding late-night or large meals, which reduces nighttime acid reflux symptoms.

4. **Enhanced Digestive Comfort:** Smaller, more frequent meals aid digestion and reduce the chance of stomach strain and acid reflux.

5. **Prevention of Complications:** By treating symptoms and lowering the risk of long-term damage, an acid reflux diet can help prevent complications such as Barrett's esophagus, esophageal strictures, and respiratory disorders.

6. **Better Dental Health:** Limiting acidic and sugary foods protects tooth enamel, promoting improved dental health, and lowering the incidence of acid reflux-related dental disorders.

7. **Weight Management:** Adopting a healthy acid reflux diet frequently incorporates elements of a balanced, nutritious diet, which aids in weight management.

8. **Optimized Nutrient Absorption:** Choosing nutrient-dense meals promotes general health and guarantees that necessary vitamins and minerals are received by the body despite dietary constraints.

9. **Enhanced Quality of Life:** Reduced acid reflux symptoms result in a higher quality of life. Individuals can go about their everyday lives without experiencing the discomfort and inconveniences that come with untreated acid reflux.

10. **Potential Reduction in Medication Dependency:** An acid reflux diet may lessen the need for certain drugs, allowing for a more natural and holistic approach to symptom management.

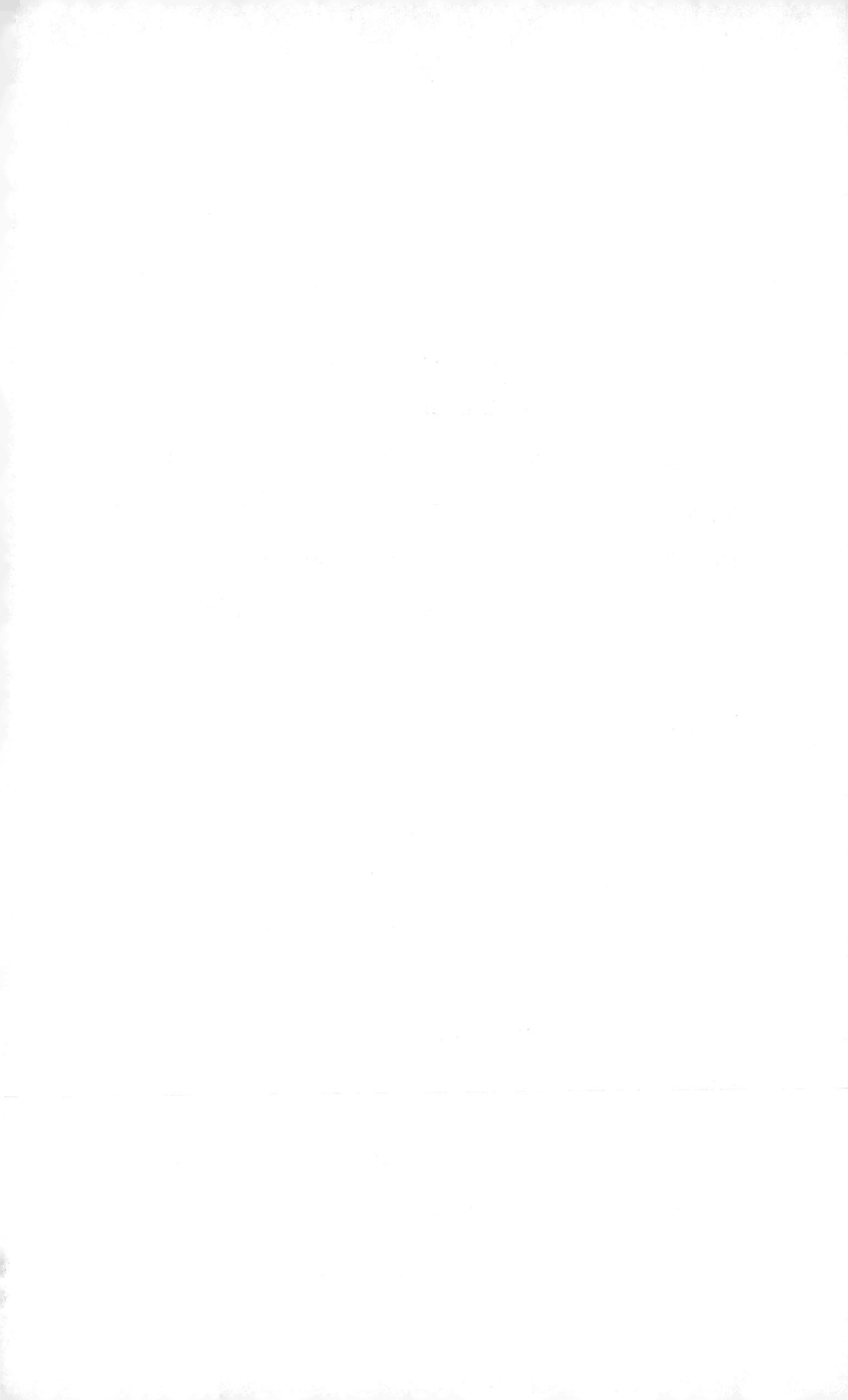

Conclusion

This cookbook is a beacon of culinary empowerment in the arena of gastronomic triumph over acid reflux. It is more than just a cookbook; it is a manifesto for recovering the joy of eating without the constraints of discomfort. Each carefully crafted recipe captures the precise mix of flavor and digestive ease, providing a road map to a life free of acid reflux restrictions.

As we embark on this culinary adventure, keep in mind that the mastery of acid reflux resides not only in pharmacological cures but also on the plate. With each dish, this cookbook transforms into a compass, directing readers toward meals that both satisfy the palette and nourish the body. It's an invitation to embark on a gastronomic adventure where nourishment meets delight and every bite is a victory.

As we say goodbye to these pages, let the kitchen become a haven of delight, a place where acidity yields to the harmonic symphony of flavors. May this cookbook be the trigger for a future when meals are savored and acid reflux is a distant memory—a life abundantly seasoned with the enjoyment of wholesome, enjoyable eating. Cheers to the art of culinary emancipation!

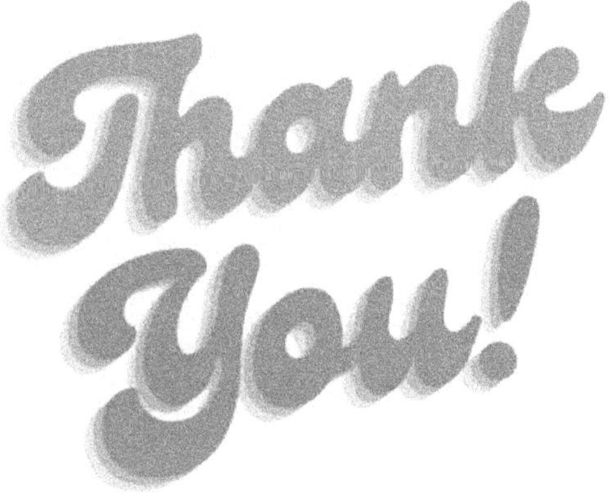

WEEKLY MEAL

JOURNAL

 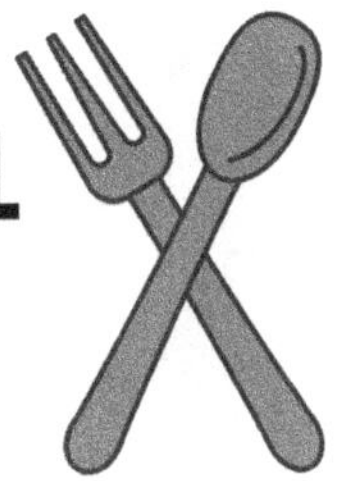

Weekly Meal Planner

Monday

Breakfast	
Lunch	
Dinner	

Tuesday

Breakfast	
Lunch	
Dinner	

Wednesday

Breakfast	
Lunch	
Dinner	

Thursday

Breakfast	
Lunch	
Dinner	

Friday

Breakfast	
Lunch	
Dinner	

Saturday

Breakfast	
Lunch	
Dinner	

Sunday

Breakfast	
Lunch	
Dinner	

Note

Weekly Meal Planner

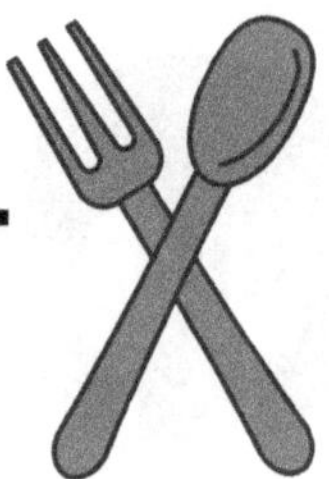

Monday

Breakfast	
Lunch	
Dinner	

Tuesday

Breakfast	
Lunch	
Dinner	

Wednesday

Breakfast	
Lunch	
Dinner	

Thursday

Breakfast	
Lunch	
Dinner	

Friday

Breakfast	
Lunch	
Dinner	

Saturday

Breakfast	
Lunch	
Dinner	

Sunday

Breakfast	
Lunch	
Dinner	

Note

Weekly Meal Planner

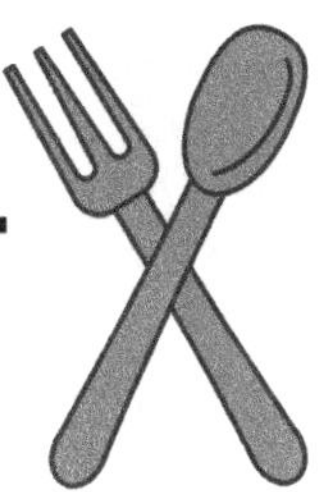

Monday

Breakfast	
Lunch	
Dinner	

Tuesday

Breakfast	
Lunch	
Dinner	

Wednesday

Breakfast	
Lunch	
Dinner	

Thursday

Breakfast	
Lunch	
Dinner	

Friday

Breakfast	
Lunch	
Dinner	

Saturday

Breakfast	
Lunch	
Dinner	

Sunday

Breakfast	
Lunch	
Dinner	

Note

Weekly Meal Planner

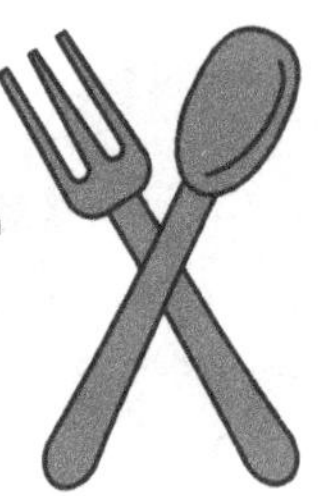

Monday

Breakfast	
Lunch	
Dinner	

Tuesday

Breakfast	
Lunch	
Dinner	

Wednesday

Breakfast	
Lunch	
Dinner	

Thursday

Breakfast	
Lunch	
Dinner	

Friday

Breakfast	
Lunch	
Dinner	

Saturday

Breakfast	
Lunch	
Dinner	

Sunday

Breakfast	
Lunch	
Dinner	

Note

Weekly Meal Planner

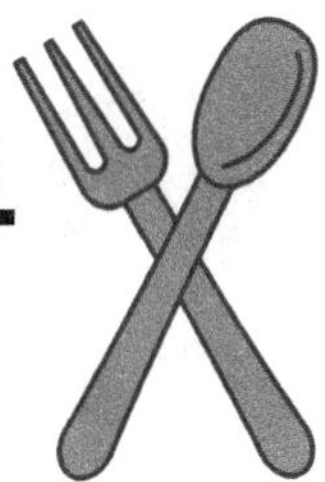

Monday

Breakfast	
Lunch	
Dinner	

Tuesday

Breakfast	
Lunch	
Dinner	

Wednesday

Breakfast	
Lunch	
Dinner	

Thursday

Breakfast	
Lunch	
Dinner	

Friday

Breakfast	
Lunch	
Dinner	

Saturday

Breakfast	
Lunch	
Dinner	

Sunday

Breakfast	
Lunch	
Dinner	

Note

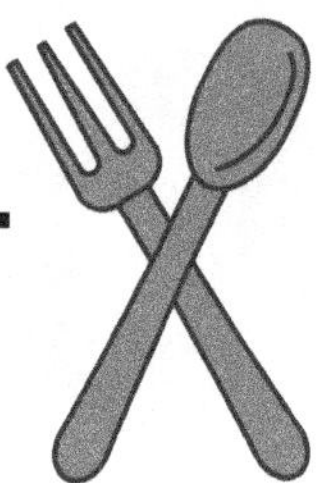

Weekly Meal Planner

Monday

Breakfast	
Lunch	
Dinner	

Tuesday

Breakfast	
Lunch	
Dinner	

Wednesday

Breakfast	
Lunch	
Dinner	

Thursday

Breakfast	
Lunch	
Dinner	

Friday

Breakfast	
Lunch	
Dinner	

Saturday

Breakfast	
Lunch	
Dinner	

Sunday

Breakfast	
Lunch	
Dinner	

Note

 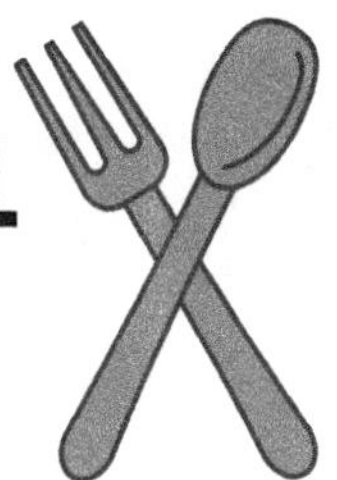

Weekly Meal Planner

Monday

Breakfast	
Lunch	
Dinner	

Tuesday

Breakfast	
Lunch	
Dinner	

Wednesday

Breakfast	
Lunch	
Dinner	

Thursday

Breakfast	
Lunch	
Dinner	

Friday

Breakfast	
Lunch	
Dinner	

Saturday

Breakfast	
Lunch	
Dinner	

Sunday

Breakfast	
Lunch	
Dinner	

Note

 # Weekly Meal Planner 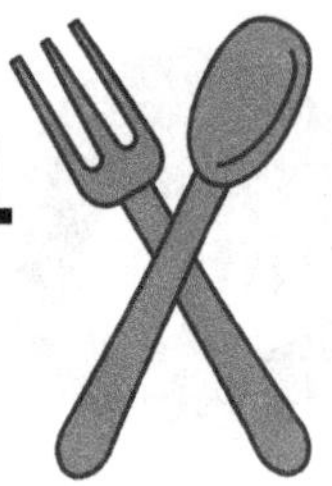

Monday

Breakfast	
Lunch	
Dinner	

Tuesday

Breakfast	
Lunch	
Dinner	

Wednesday

Breakfast	
Lunch	
Dinner	

Thursday

Breakfast	
Lunch	
Dinner	

Friday

Breakfast	
Lunch	
Dinner	

Saturday

Breakfast	
Lunch	
Dinner	

Sunday

Breakfast	
Lunch	
Dinner	

Note

 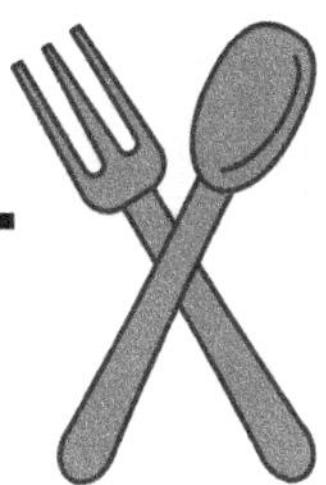

Weekly Meal Planner

Monday

Breakfast	
Lunch	
Dinner	

Tuesday

Breakfast	
Lunch	
Dinner	

Wednesday

Breakfast	
Lunch	
Dinner	

Thursday

Breakfast	
Lunch	
Dinner	

Friday

Breakfast	
Lunch	
Dinner	

Saturday

Breakfast	
Lunch	
Dinner	

Sunday

Breakfast	
Lunch	
Dinner	

Note

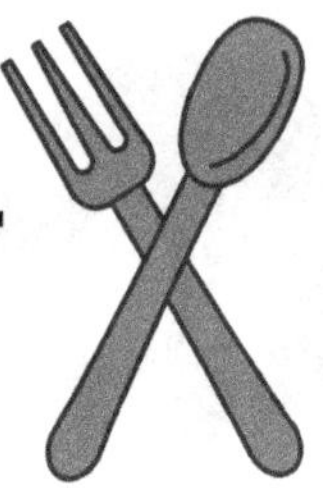

Weekly Meal Planner

Monday

Breakfast	
Lunch	
Dinner	

Tuesday

Breakfast	
Lunch	
Dinner	

Wednesday

Breakfast	
Lunch	
Dinner	

Thursday

Breakfast	
Lunch	
Dinner	

Friday

Breakfast	
Lunch	
Dinner	

Saturday

Breakfast	
Lunch	
Dinner	

Sunday

Breakfast	
Lunch	
Dinner	

Note

 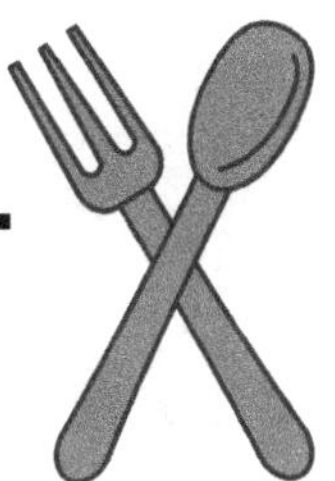

Weekly Meal Planner

Monday

Breakfast	
Lunch	
Dinner	

Tuesday

Breakfast	
Lunch	
Dinner	

Wednesday

Breakfast	
Lunch	
Dinner	

Thursday

Breakfast	
Lunch	
Dinner	

Friday

Breakfast	
Lunch	
Dinner	

Saturday

Breakfast	
Lunch	
Dinner	

Sunday

Breakfast	
Lunch	
Dinner	

Note

Weekly Meal Planner

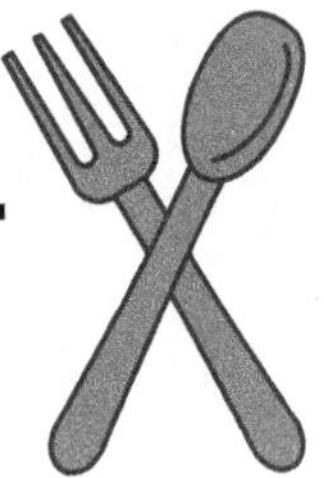

Monday

Breakfast	
Lunch	
Dinner	

Tuesday

Breakfast	
Lunch	
Dinner	

Wednesday

Breakfast	
Lunch	
Dinner	

Thursday

Breakfast	
Lunch	
Dinner	

Friday

Breakfast	
Lunch	
Dinner	

Saturday

Breakfast	
Lunch	
Dinner	

Sunday

Breakfast	
Lunch	
Dinner	

Note

 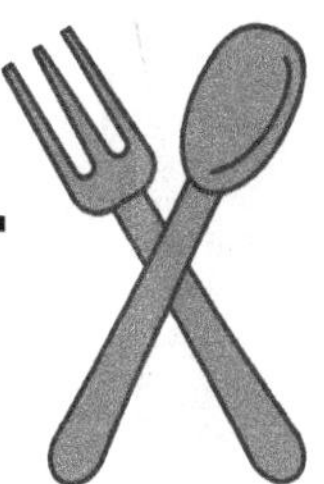

Weekly Meal Planner

Monday

Breakfast	
Lunch	
Dinner	

Tuesday

Breakfast	
Lunch	
Dinner	

Wednesday

Breakfast	
Lunch	
Dinner	

Thursday

Breakfast	
Lunch	
Dinner	

Friday

Breakfast	
Lunch	
Dinner	

Saturday

Breakfast	
Lunch	
Dinner	

Sunday

Breakfast	
Lunch	
Dinner	

Note

Weekly Meal Planner

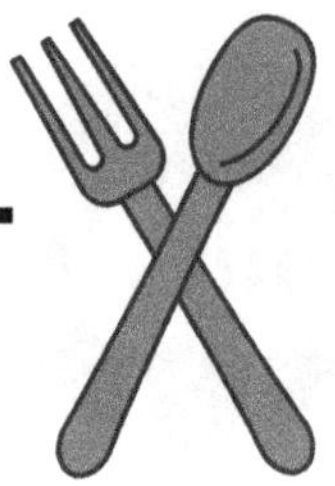

Monday

Breakfast	
Lunch	
Dinner	

Tuesday

Breakfast	
Lunch	
Dinner	

Wednesday

Breakfast	
Lunch	
Dinner	

Thursday

Breakfast	
Lunch	
Dinner	

Friday

Breakfast	
Lunch	
Dinner	

Saturday

Breakfast	
Lunch	
Dinner	

Sunday

Breakfast	
Lunch	
Dinner	

Note

 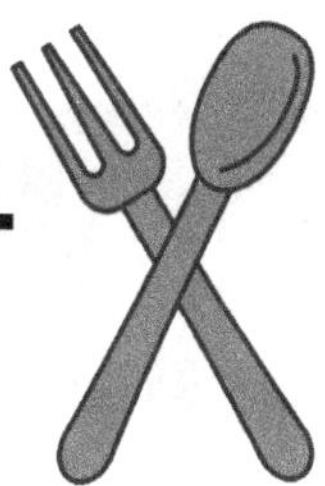

Weekly Meal Planner

Monday

Breakfast	
Lunch	
Dinner	

Tuesday

Breakfast	
Lunch	
Dinner	

Wednesday

Breakfast	
Lunch	
Dinner	

Thursday

Breakfast	
Lunch	
Dinner	

Friday

Breakfast	
Lunch	
Dinner	

Saturday

Breakfast	
Lunch	
Dinner	

Sunday

Breakfast	
Lunch	
Dinner	

Note

 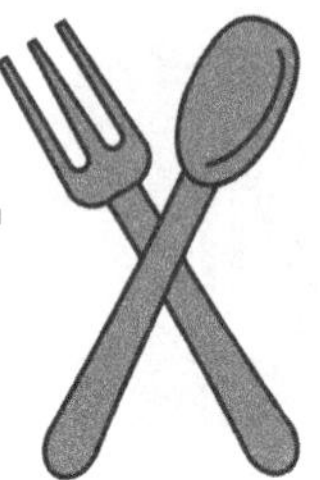

Weekly Meal Planner

Monday

Breakfast	
Lunch	
Dinner	

Tuesday

Breakfast	
Lunch	
Dinner	

Wednesday

Breakfast	
Lunch	
Dinner	

Thursday

Breakfast	
Lunch	
Dinner	

Friday

Breakfast	
Lunch	
Dinner	

Saturday

Breakfast	
Lunch	
Dinner	

Sunday

Breakfast	
Lunch	
Dinner	

Note

www.ingramcontent.com/pod-product-compliance
Lightning Source LLC
Chambersburg PA
CBHW071610270726
48661CB00019B/1943